Proof That Face Masks Do More Harm Than Good

Dr Vernon Coleman MB ChB DSc
Sunday Times Bestselling Author

This short book contains conclusive proof that face masks do more harm than good, and being forced to wear them is a form of oppression designed to have adverse physical and psychological effects upon the wearer rather than having any protective value.

A Thank You Note

My sincere thanks go to all those who have supported and encouraged my fight to share the truth about the coronavirus hoax. You are too numerous to mention by name but my thanks to you all.

'Those who would give up essential liberty, to purchase a little temporary safety, deserve neither liberty nor safety.'
Benjamin Franklin

Table of Contents

Introduction

To my horror and disappointment the shops, and indeed
the streets, are full of mask-wearing muppets. In the
shops everything takes an age as shopper and assistant
struggle to make themselves heard through their masks.
The muppets have become mumblies.
Many mask wearers keep their masks on even when out
of doors, where it is not yet mandatory to do so. These
over-compliant collaborators are making oppression easy
for the totalitarians who will doubtless soon be
demanding that we all wear our masks wherever we are
and whatever we are doing – even in our own homes.
Most mask wearers have no idea of the harm they are
doing by wearing masks. Indeed, many seem to
understand very little about how to wear a mask. I have,
on several occasions, seen people drop their mask onto
the pavement – face side down of course – pick it up and
put it on. Many people wear the same mask for more
than two hours (which is dangerous), wear disposable
masks more than once (which is dangerous), fail to wash
cloth masks (which means they accumulate bacteria,
fungi and viruses – all of which are breathed in) touch
their mask while it is in position (which makes the mask
even worse than useless), put masks into their pockets or
handbags and then put them back on creased and grubby
(a very dangerous thing to do since the wearer will then
be breathing in whatever bugs have been transmitted to
the mask. Scarves are often used as face coverings
without ever being washed (an effective way to catch
throat and lung infections). Nearly everyone constantly

fiddles with their masks – not realising that touching a mask is something you should not do. The incidence of throat and chest infections is going to rocket. I wonder how many people will be killed by their masks. We'll never know.

What the hell has happened to people? I am appalled at how easily people have become so compliant and have accepted the Government lies. Many mask wearers now choose their masks as fashion items and wear masks designed to match their outfits. A few wear dark glasses and gloves as well as masks. I fear they probably think they look cool and well-dressed.

As I said earlier, it won't be long before the Government will order people to wear masks in the home. And they will. Some will sleep in them – and doubtless die in them.

Most mask wearers are clearly being made ill by their masks. Because their oxygen levels are low, their eyes are glazed, as though they are drugged.

When the covid-19 hoax began, authorities around the world announced that mask wearing was pointless, and it was widely agreed by experts that they could probably do more harm than good. Indeed, mask wearing was dismissed as 'virtue signalling' by Dr Fauci, the American coronavirus expert. The World Health Organisation supported this general view which was in accordance with the available scientific evidence. Medical advisors around the world agreed that there was no need to wear masks.

Later during the year, the story changed.

Although there did not seem to be any scientific evidence supporting such a dramatic change, the World Health Organisation suddenly supported face mask wearing. Almost instantly, governments around the world, led by medical and scientific advisors, changed their views overnight and decided that we should all wear masks. The WHO's main financial supporter is the American software billionaire Bill Gates who has a number of powerful alliances with media organisations (such as the BBC), strong financial links with Monsanto and a number of drug companies, and an enthusiasm for vaccination which, to put it politely, does not seem justified by the evidence.

Why, in the absence of a change in medical advice did the WHO change its mind?

Well, it seems that the campaign for masks to be worn worldwide was either founded by the World Economic Forum, which advocates a global reset and of which that well-known 'medical expert' Prince Charles of England appears to be a leading member, or by an organisation called masks4all. The promotion of masks was supported by Goldman Sachs, the bank, in my view one of the most evil companies on earth (along with Google and Monsanto) which was once memorably described by Matt Taibbi as a vampire squid on the face of humanity. The bank is reported to have claimed that if everyone in America wore a mask, the American economy would be boosted.

I have no idea how they came to this conclusion or why they think their advice is better than medical research.

The masks4all website promotes the slogan, 'Anyone without a mask puts you and your family at risk', and masks4all is a fiscally sponsored project of something called Community Initiatives which seems to have links to a whole range of organisations I've never heard of. As a result of the WHO's change of advice, media throughout the world also changed their advice. The well-known video sharing site called YouTube betrayed users by deleting videos made by doctors (such as myself) which offered scientific evidence proving that masks are of no value but are dangerous.

I could find no convincing scientific evidence supporting this change of heart but, as a result of the WHO's about-turn, populations everywhere were forced to wear masks – or to risk being fined. Only those prepared to self-certify that they could not wear a mask were allowed to travel on trains or buses or any other form of public transport without a face covering. And shortly afterwards, the rule was extended to cover shops and public buildings. Strangely, people in offices were not always forced to wear masks – as though the coronavirus were in some way inactive in a working environment but active in a shopping environment.

I have kept this book short and have resisted the mild temptation to include a history of mask wearing in all its various forms. The only thing that is important at the moment is whether mask wearing is useful and necessary or dangerous and being forced upon us as part of the new totalitarianism.

I repeat, I have yet to find any reliable scientific evidence proving that masks are useful, safe or worth wearing. Many doctors who are not employed by governments or public agencies, seem to agree that mask wearing is very likely to do far more harm than good. The available scientific evidence shows that masks, whatever their form, provide a poor obstacle to infective organisms but do impede air intake and oxygen exchange.

Those who wear masks are collaborating in a massive conspiracy.

Important Note: My first video in March 2020 was entitled, *Coronavirus Scare – the Hoax of the Century?*. What I meant by this, and have subsequently made clear on many occasions, is not that the existence of covid-19 itself is a hoax, but that the exaggerated, fraudulent response was unnecessary, harmful and deliberately designed to over-sell a not unusual seasonal virus infection. The covid-19 infection is merely a standard flu heavily marketed for a specific purpose: the lockdowns, the social distancing, the masks, and the vaccines were never necessary, and it is not difficult to prove that these measures have done infinitely more harm than good and will, in due course, result in far more deaths than covid-19.

If this really were a pandemic, there would have been no need for governments to fiddle the covid death figures. For example, if someone dies within 28 or 60 days of having had a positive PCR test (a test that is known to have a high rate of false positives) then that person is automatically put down as a covid death. That is fraud. It is not unknown for the ordinary flu to kill 650,000 people globally in a single, six month flu season but today the flu has virtually disappeared but the mainstream media appears to have failed to make this pretty obvious connection.

There would have been no need for governments and the media to lie, lie and lie again. And, most important of all, there would have been no need to silence, suppress and demonise all those wishing to question the officially promoted lies. Never, in history, has medical debate been so effectively oppressed and doctors wishing to share simple truths been so ruthlessly silenced. It is also worth remembering that many of the so-called fact checkers are nothing of the sort. There are now hundreds of self-acclaimed fact checkers around the world, and many of them receive huge donations from individuals, corporations and charities with views and vested interests to protect. Many of the fact checkers seem to be employed largely to suppress the truth and to discredit those who are sharing the truth.

The day after my first video appeared on YouTube, my Wikipedia page was changed dramatically to discredit me. And shortly after that, the video was removed. Subsequently, hundreds of videos made by myself and other independent doctors have been removed though the views of pro-establishment celebrities, with no medical knowledge or understanding, have been promoted vigorously. Anyone who wants to know why all this has happened will find the answers in my book, *Endgame: The Hidden Agenda 21*.

Masks and Mask Wearing: 111 Facts You Must Know

1.

Surgeons have been using surgical masks since their introduction in 1897. It has for some years been customary for surgeons and nurses to wear surgical masks in the operating theatre and to change masks part of the way through any procedure lasting more than a few hours.

The dangers associated with mask wearing were assessed by five doctors and published in the journal *Neurocirugia* in 2008.

Although it is customary for operating theatres to be fitted with air conditioning systems, the writers of the article, entitled, *Preliminary Report on Surgical Mask induced Deoxygenation During Major Surgery*, pointed out that it is known that heat and moisture are trapped beneath surgical masks and concluded that 'it seems reasonable that some of the exhaled carbon dioxide may also be trapped beneath them, inducing a decrease in blood oxygenation'.

A total of 53 surgeons, of both sexes, all employed at university hospitals and aged between 24 and 54 years of age were tested. All were non-smokers and none had any chronic lung disease. The test involved pulse oximetry before and after the course of an operation. The study showed that the longer a mask was worn the greater the fall in blood oxygen levels. This may lead to the individual passing out and it may also affect natural immunity – thereby increasing the risk of infection.

The masks used were disposable, sterile, one-way surgical paper masks. To eliminate the effect of dehydration over a several hour surgical operation, the surgeons were allowed after every hour to drink water through a straw.

The authors of the paper concluded that, 'When the values for oxygen saturation of haemoglobin were compared, there were statistically significant differences only between preoperational and post operational values. As the duration of the operation increases, oxygen saturation of haemoglobin decreases significantly.'

2.

This quote is taken from *New England Journal of Medicine*: 'We know that wearing a mask outside health care facilities offers little, if any, protection from infection. Public health authorities define a significant exposure to covid-19 as face to face contact within six feet with a patient with symptomatic covid-19 that is sustained for at least a few minutes (and some say more than 10 minutes or even 20 minutes). The chance of catching covid-19 from a passing interaction in a public space is therefore minimal. In many cases the desire for widespread masking is a reflexive reaction to anxiety over the pandemic.' The reference: M. Klompas, C. Morris et al 'Universal Masking in hospitals in the covid-19 era' – *New England Journal of Medicine 2020*

3.

It is possible that wearing a mask for hours at a time could cause pulmonary fibrosis. In August 1988, the proceedings of the VIIth International Pneumoconioses Conference included details of three cases of pulmonary fibrosis, thought to be due to exposure to synthetic textile fibres. The first was a woman of 52 who had a dry cough with increasing difficulty in breathing. Changes were visible on an X-ray. The woman had been working in a textile shop for 15 years where her job was measuring and cutting cloth – mainly synthetic materials. The second patient was a woman of 66 who also had difficulty in breathing. The lungs of this patient also showed X-ray changes. She was also involved in cutting and measuring synthetic fabrics. A third woman, aged 47, had bilateral pulmonary fibrosis. Studies have shown that loose fibres are seen on all types of masks and may be inhaled causing serious lung damage.

4.

People who cough and sneeze into their mask increase the risk of a build-up of fungi and bacteria – which can lead to dangerous chest infections.

5.

In 2015, the *British Medical Journal* published a paper entitled, *A Cluster Randomised Trial of Cloth Masks Compared with Medical Masks in Healthcare Workers*. The paper was written by nine authors from the University of New South Wales, the University of Sydney, the National Institute of Hygiene and Epidemiology in Vietnam and the Beijing Centers for Disease Control and Prevention in China. The aim of the study was to compare the efficacy of cloth masks to medical masks in hospital health care workers. The study, which was extensive, concluded that the results caution against the use of cloth masks.

'This is an important finding to inform occupational health and safety,' concluded the authors. 'Moisture retention, reuse of cloth masks and poor filtration may result in increased risk of infection.'

And the authors added: '…as a precautionary measure, cloth masks should not be recommended for health care workers, particularly in high risk situations, and guidelines need to be updated'.

6.

Many individuals have turned their masks into fashion items. I wonder how many wear the same mask day after day without washing them. If masks are unwashed then they become breeding grounds for bacteria, fungi and viruses. If they are washed then they become even more useless (if that is possible) than they were when new. The enthusiasm for 'fashion' masks, which match other items of clothing, is rising. But wearing a fashionable mask is akin to a slave painting their chains to look pretty.

7.

The word 'covering' is now often used in official propaganda material, having replaced the word 'mask'. It has clearly been decreed more acceptable than the more usual word 'mask' which carries worrying overtones.

8.

It is often difficult to hear what people say when they are wearing masks – particularly if the masks are close-fitting. Conversations are kept to a minimum and social interactions in shops and other establishments are functional at best. (It is worth noting that hairdressers and others in service industries have been instructed to talk as little as possible – ostensibly to prevent the spread of the virus. Also, singing, a joyful activity for singers and listeners, has been banned.)

9.

Mask wearers have been encouraged by the psy-op specialists employed by governments to show their hatred for non-mask wearers. This loathsome ploy was first promoted by Ms Dick of the Metropolitan police in London, and seems designed to make those who cannot or do not wear masks feel guilty and ashamed. The mentally and physically disabled will, therefore, be harassed and abused if they dare to go out of their homes.

10.

In October 2020, it was noticeable that when street photographs were published in the press or online, they invariably showed members of the public wearing masks – even though mask wearing out of doors was not compulsory. Were the public being conditioned for the time that wearing masks outdoors becomes mandatory?

11.

Symptoms caused by mask wearing are now being wrongly blamed on covid-19. It seems likely that when mask wearing starts to result in deaths (as it will do), those deaths will be blamed on covid-19 and used as a reason for politicians and advisors to demand that people wear masks for even longer hours. The vicious circle will be complete.

12.

The Occupational Safety and Health Administration in the US has decreed that any room where the carbon dioxide is present at a level or more than 5,000 parts per million is unsafe and has an environment which is toxic and dangerous. Carbon dioxide levels normally exist at between 350 and 450 parts per million. Acceptable indoor quality level is 600 to 800 ppm. Any employer who attempts to force employees to work in an environment where the carbon dioxide level is too high can be held to account. Similarly, any teacher who attempts to force children to study in such an environment would be legally responsible. If a nuclear submarine has a level of over 5,000 parts per million then it must surface because it is considered to have a threatening and dangerous environment. There is much dispute about the levels of carbon dioxide which may develop if a mask is worn. Generally, the tighter a mask fits the greater the risk that the level of carbon dioxide will rise to dangerous levels but it must be remembered that most members of the public have no training on how to wear a mask and there are few if any restrictions on mask manufacture. Indeed, members of the public are making their own masks and using bits of left over material to do so. A wide variety of masks are being designed and worn. Those dismissing the danger as non-existent might like to read HSE Contract Research Report no 27/1991, produced by the British Health and Safety Executive and entitled, *Dead space and inhaled carbon dioxide levels in respiratory protective equipment*. Those dismissing the risks associated with carbon dioxide levels should know that the amount of carbon dioxide in a small room can easily rise to levels which are dangerous enough to have a dramatic effect on decision making. At least eight studies in the last decade have studied carbon dioxide levels indoors and have found worrying levels above 1,200 parts per million.

13.

Women giving birth in France have to wear face masks. In my opinion, this is dangerous and will put extra strain on the heart. Pregnant women should not wear a mask, not only because of the risk to themselves but because of the risk to their unborn child. There is a real risk that the baby will be stillborn or in some way damaged or poorly developed at birth.

14.

Research conducted by four French doctors in 2018 and reported in *Rev Mal Respir*, was designed to evaluate the effect of wearing a surgical mask during a six minute walking test. The authors of the study were E. Person, C.

Lemercier, A. Royer and G. Reychler. (The six minute walking test is regularly used in pulmonology.)

For this research, 44 health subjects were used. Each individual performed two six minute walking tests – one with a mask and one without a mask.

The researchers found that dyspnoea variation was significantly higher with a surgical mask, and concluded that the difference was clinically relevant.

The conclusion was that 'wearing a surgical mask modifies significantly and clinically dyspnoea.'

15.

Mask wearers, of a sanctimonious nature, will sometimes claim that they wear masks not to protect themselves but to protect other people. This is simple-minded nonsense since, as has been well demonstrated in this book, face masks are of no value to anyone and, indeed, can be a menace both to those wearing them and to those maskless people they meet.

16.

Vital evidence outlining the dangers and ineffectiveness of mask wearing has been banned, blocked or deleted from the internet. Videos assessing the value of wearing face masks on the basis of the scientific evidence have been removed. Discussion and debate about the value of face masks are suppressed by politicians and the media. Research material outlining the dangers of mask wearing has been removed from the internet on the basis that 'it is no longer relevant in our current climate'. So-called 'fact-checkers' invariably dismiss medical reports published by doctors and scientists – however eminent those experts might be. The so-called 'fact-checkers' are often linked to commercial organisations or groups with commercial links. No one seems to check the 'fact-checkers' – though they should.

17.
Between 2004 and 2016, at least twelve articles appeared in medical and scientific journals showing that face masks do not prevent the transmission of infection.

18.
There are no strict rules about what constitutes a face mask, and the rules about when and where masks should be worn are constantly changing. This proves that there is no science supporting the wearing of masks. So, for example, it is clearly absurd that the coronavirus should be thought to spread from person to person in a shop but not in an office.

19.
The tighter a mask fits the more likely it is to reduce blood oxygen levels and to increase the amount of carbon dioxide being inhaled. It should be noted that optimal oxygen intake in humans should, according to the US Occupational Safety and Health Administration, be between 19.5 and 23.5% and that any human-occupied airspace where oxygen measures less than 19.5% should be labelled as not safe for workers. However, the percentage of oxygen inside a masked airspace generally measures 17.4% within seconds of

putting on the mask. A tighter fitting mask will result in lower oxygen levels and higher carbon dioxide levels. Lower oxygen levels and increased levels of carbon dioxide stimulate greater inspiratory flow – leading to a greater risk that loose fibres from the face mask will be inhaled.

20.

In Belgium, in September 2020, a group of 70 doctors sent an open letter to Ben Weyts, the Flemish Education Minister in which they claimed that children are badly affected by having to wear face masks. 'Mandatory face masks in schools are a major threat to their development,' they wrote. 'It ignores the essential need of the growing child. The well-being of children and young people is highly dependent on emotional attachment to others.'

(Observing facial expressions help a child's social development and so seeing those around them wearing masks must therefore delay a child's development.)

According to *The Brussels Times*, the doctors continued that 'there is no large-scale evidence that wearing face masks in a non-professional environment has any positive effect on the spread of viruses, let alone on general health. Nor is there any legal basis for implementing this requirement.'

'Meanwhile, it is clear that healthy children living through covid-19 heal without complications as standard and that they subsequently contribute to the protection of their fellow human beings by increasing group immunity.'

'The only sensible measure to prevent serious illness and mortality caused by covid-19 is to isolate individual teachers and individual children at increased risk,' they added. 'This risk assessment is not the task of the Ministry of Education but the task of the treating physicians in consultation with their patients.'

21.
Leading German virologist Professor Streeck has criticised the use of masks, which he has said are a wonderful breeding ground for bacteria and fungi. He has also criticised lockdowns.

22.
Two dentists in New York have reported seeing a number of patients with inflamed gums and other problems. The news story was reported in the *New York Post*.
'We're seeing inflammation in people's gums that have been healthy forever, and cavities in people who have never had them before,' said dentist Rob Ramondi.
'About 50% of our patients are being impacted by this, (so) we decided to name it 'mask mouth'.'
Another dentist, Marc Sclafani, told the *New York Post* that 'gum disease, or periodontal disease, will eventually lead to strokes and an increased risk of heart attacks.'
The dentists said that the problem is caused by the fact that face coverings increase mouth dryness and contribute to a build-up of bad bacteria.
'People tend to breathe through their mouth instead of through their nose while wearing a mask,' said Sclafani.

'The mouth breathing is causing the dry mouth, which leads to a decrease in saliva – and saliva is what fights the bacteria and cleanses your teeth.'

23.
Masks diminish the quality of our relationships with other people. We trust people less if they are wearing masks. We cannot see smiles and so we fear people more.

24.
When the truth finally comes out about the dangers of masks, teachers making children wear masks in schools will be sued. Bosses making their employees wear masks will also be sued. Ignorance is no defence. And as the Nuremburg defendants discovered, the reply 'I was obeying orders' is no defence.

25.
A 26-year-old man suffered a collapsed lung after running 2.5 miles while wearing a face mask. Doctors say his condition was caused by the high pressure on the man's lung due to his intense breathing while wearing the face mask. When masks are made mandatory outdoors in the UK, joggers and cyclists will have no choice but to wear masks. Many will die.

26.
Never in history have so many people worn masks obstructing their intake of air. A considerable amount of research has been done into mask wearing. The research

shows clearly that masks are ineffective in preventing the movement of infective organisms but that they reduce oxygen levels and increase levels of carbon dioxide. Most of those advocating mask wearing are either ignorant or are deliberately exposing mask wearers to danger. The side effects of excess carbon dioxide (hypercapnia) are headaches, dizziness, drowsiness, nausea, vomiting and a tight feeling in the chest. The risks are usually dismissed as irrelevant or non-existent by government spokesmen and fact checkers (many of whom are sponsored by industry) but I found it impossible to find reliable scientific evidence supporting this reassurance. It should be noted that the BBC, which claims to produce fact checking material, has financial links to the Bill and Melinda Gates Foundation (which itself has strong financial links to the vaccine industry among others) and is in my view entirely untrustworthy. The question, as always, is a simple one: who will check the 'fact checkers'?

Government defenders regard the removal of a video from YouTube as a sign that the advice in the video must have been 'wrong'. The reality, of course, is the exact opposite since YouTube takes down material which disagrees with advice from the World Health Organisation which is now heavily sponsored by the Bill and Melinda Gates Foundation.

27.

Streets are littered with discarded face masks which ought to have been incinerated as medical waste, if this really were a highly dangerous virus. It is important to note that, on March 19th 2020, the public health bodies and the Advisory Committee on Dangerous Pathogens decided that covid-19 should no longer be classified as a 'high consequence infectious disease' – the link for the proof of this is on my website www.vernoncoleman.com. A couple of days after this decision, the UK Government introduced lockdowns and introduced the most oppressive Bill in British Parliamentary history.

28.

It was reported in *The Sydney Morning Herald* in 2003, that retailers who cash in on community fears about SARS by exaggerating the health benefits of surgical masks could face fines of up to $110,000. NSW Fair Trading Minister Reba Meagher warned that distributors and traders could be prosecuted if it was suggested the masks offered unrealistic levels of protection from the disease. 'There appears to be some debate about whether surgical masks are able to minimise the effects of SARS.' Ms Meagher said her department would investigate any complaints about false mask claims which concerned the public.

Health authorities have warned that surgical masks may not be an effective protection against the virus. 'Those masks are only effective so long as they are dry,' said Professor Yvonne Cossart of the Department of Infectious Disease at the University of Sydney. 'As soon as they become saturated with moisture in your breath they stop doing their job and pass on the droplets.' Professor Cossart said that could take as little as 15 or 20 minutes, after which the mask would need to be changed.'

29.
Does wearing a face mask reduce your immunity levels? No one seems to know the answer for sure but it seems possible that if people wear face masks for long periods (months or years) then the absence of contact with the real world might well have a harmful effect on immunity – if the face mask works. Do face masks prevent us developing immunity to particular diseases? This depends on many factors – mainly the effectiveness of the face mask. But if the mask isn't preventing the development of immunity then it probably isn't worth wearing anyway.

30.
It is widely acknowledged that wearing a face mask may give a false sense of security and may stop the wearer taking other precautions – such as washing their hands. Also, it has been established that if masks aren't worn properly, and changed regularly, they can do much more harm than good.

31.
There is no doubt that face masks can be dangerous. In China, two school boys who were wearing face masks while running on a track both collapsed and died – possibly, I would surmise, because the strain on their hearts by the shortage of oxygen proved fatal. According to the German doctor, Dr Bodo Schiffmann, at least three

other children may have died in Germany due to mask wearing.

32.

A report published in the *British Medical Journal* summarised some other risks. First, when you wear a face mask some of the air you breathe out goes into your eyes. This can be annoying and uncomfortable and if, as a result, you touch your eyes you may infect yourself. Second, face masks make breathing more difficult and, as I have already pointed out, anyone who has a breathing problem will find that a mask makes it worse. Also, some of the carbon dioxide which is breathed out with each exhalation is then breathed in because it is trapped. Together these factors may mean that the mask wearer may breathe more frequently or more deeply, and if that happens then someone who has the coronavirus may end up breathing more of the virus into their lungs. If a mask is contaminated because it has been worn for too long then the risks are even greater. How long is too long? No one knows but two hours seems an accepted limit. No research has been done as far as I know. Third, there is a risk that the accumulation of the virus in the fabric of the mask may increase the amount of the virus being breathed in. This might then defeat the body's immune response and cause an increase in infections – other infections, not just the coronavirus.

33.

Dr Russell Blaylock, a retired neurosurgeon, has reported that wearing a face mask can produce a number of problems varying from headaches to hypercapnia (a condition in which excess carbon dioxide accumulates in the body) and that the problems can include life-threatening complications. Symptoms of hypercapnia include drowsiness, dizziness and fatigue. Some of the carbon dioxide exhaled with each breath is retained behind the mask and then breathed in again.

Dr Blaylock has also warned of neurological problems. 'By wearing a mask, the exhaled viruses will not be able to escape and will concentrate in the nasal passages, enter the olfactory nerves and travel into the brain,' he wrote.

And Dr Blaylock has warned of the danger to patients with cancer. 'People with cancer, especially if the cancer has spread, will be at a further risk from prolonged hypoxia as the cancer grows best in a microenvironment that is low in oxygen. Low oxygen also promotes inflammation which can promote the growth, invasion and spread of cancers. Repeated episodes of hypoxia have been proposed as a significant factor in atherosclerosis and hence increases (the risk of) all cardiovascular and cerebrovascular diseases.'

34.

The risk of side effects developing when wearing a mask depend to some extent on whether the mask is made of cloth or paper or is an N95 mask filtering out at least 95% of airborne particles. One study of 212 healthcare workers showed that a third of them developed headaches with 60% needing painkillers to relieve the headache. Some of the headaches were thought to be caused by an increase in the amount of carbon dioxide in the blood or a reduction in the amount of oxygen in the blood. Another study, this time of 159 young health workers, showed that 81% developed headaches after wearing face masks – so much so that their work was affected.

35.

An N95 mask can reduce blood oxygenation by as much as 20% and this can lead to a loss of consciousness. Naturally, this can be dangerous for vehicle drivers; masked bus drivers, for example, could be putting their passengers' lives at risk.

36.

Dr Blaylock has pointed to a study entitled, *The use of masks and respirators to prevent transmission of influenza: a systematic review of the scientific evidence.* This study looked at 17 separate studies and concluded that none of the studies established a conclusive relationship between the use of masks and protection against influenza infection. 'When a person has TB we have them wear a mask,' concluded Dr Blaylock, 'not the entire community of the non- infected.'
Dr Blaylock has also described how mask wearing can affect immunity. '...a drop in oxygen levels (hypoxia) is associated with an impairment in immunity,' he has written. 'Studies have shown that hypoxia can inhibit the type of main immune cells used to fight viral infections called the CD4+T- lymphocyte. This occurs because the hypoxia increases the level of a compound called

hypoxia inducible factor-11 (HIF-11) which inhibits T-lymphocytes and stimulates a powerful immune inhibitor cell. This sets the stage for contracting any infection, including covid-19, and making the consequences of that infection much graver. In essence, your mask may very well put you at an increased of infections and if so, having a much worse outcome.'

37.

Visors have one important advantage over masks. The evidence shows clearly that although masks are useless at preventing the spread of infection they are potentially extremely dangerous. On the other hand, although visors are just as useless as masks at preventing the spread of infection they are at least relatively free of danger and are, therefore, the face coverings of choice for those who feel the need to wear one. The fact that governments allow citizens to use visors proves beyond any shadow of doubt that the whole mask wearing scam is just that – a scam. The aim is to obtain psychological control rather than to control disease.

38.

Dr M Griesz-Brisson MD PhD is a leading European consultant neurologist and neurophysiologist. In October 2020, she warned that rebreathing our exhaled air, because of wearing masks, will create oxygen deficiency and an excess of carbon dioxide in the body. 'We know,' she said, 'that the human brain is very sensitive to oxygen deprivation. There are nerve cells in the hippocampus that cannot last longer than three minutes without oxygen.' Dr Griesz-Brisson pointed out that the acute warning symptoms of oxygen deprivation are headaches, drowsiness, dizziness, difficulty in concentration and slowing down of reaction times. The real danger is, however, that when the oxygen deprivation becomes chronic, the symptoms disappear because the body gets used to them. However, efficiency remains impaired and the damage to the brain continues. 'We know that neurodegenerative disease takes years to decades to develop. If today you forget your phone number, the breakdown in your brain would have already started two or three decades ago.'

Dr Griesz-Brisson explains that while the mask wearer thinks that they are becoming accustomed to re-breathing exhaled air, the problems within the brain are growing as the oxygen deprivation continues.

She also points out that brain cells which die, because of a shortage of oxygen, will never be replaced. They are gone for ever. She goes on to argue that everyone is entitled to claim exemption from mask wearing because oxygen deprivation is so dangerous – and masks don't work.

Finally, Dr Griesz-Brisson points out that children and teenagers must never wear masks, partly because they have extremely active and adaptive immune systems but also because their brains are especially active and vulnerable. The more active an organ is the more oxygen it needs. And so the damage to children's brains is huge and irreversible.

She warns that dementia is going to increase in ten years, and the younger generation will not be able to reach their potential because of the mask wearing.

Oxygen deprivation adversely affects the heart and the lungs but it also damages the brain. And the damage will be permanent.

'My conclusion has to be that no one has the right to force us to deprive our bodies of oxygen for absolutely no good reason. Depriving individuals of oxygen is a crime perpetrated by those demanding that we wear masks. Those who let it happen and those who collaborate are also guilty. And those who wear masks in situations where they are not legally required are cooperating in a criminal activity.'

Inevitably, Dr Griesz-Brisson's interview was removed from YouTube as part of the global suppression of medical information.

39.

The nasal flu vaccine, the one given to children, contains attenuated or weakened live viruses. It is possible that if a child has a weakened immune system – as would doubtless be the case if they'd been imprisoned and kept indoors a lot or had for absolutely no good reason been wearing a mask for a long time – then the attenuated virus in the vaccine might cause the flu. Because attenuated viruses aren't quite dead, they could change or even become live and they could mutate and they could result in other people being infected. So it is possible that a child who has the nasal flu vaccine could transmit the flu virus to Granny – who might die as a result.

40.

Many doctors now believe that masks are being used as a conditioning tool to make us more compliant. Most people dutifully wear them, wrongly believing that their masks will protect them from the coronavirus, and without any idea of the damage that is being done to their physical and mental health. All around the world citizens have proved to be extraordinarily obedient and gullible, pathetic even, accepting the lies and deceits quite freely. Social distancing and the wearing of masks are both likely to be long-term and possibly permanent, and the physical and mental damage done is also likely to be long-term and permanent.

41.

The rules about mask wearing change from time to time and from one area to another (proving that there is no science behind mask wearing) and we never quite know what punishments to expect. In one part of America you could be sent to prison for a year if you failed to wear a mask. In another part of America you had to pay a 2,000 dollar fine but there was no prison sentence. In Texas, some people have been told that they should wear masks in their own homes. In one shop a guard pulled a gun on a man who was not wearing a mask.

42.

The Chinese wear masks routinely – to protect themselves from pollution. But the masks appeared to make no difference to the spread of the coronavirus in China.

43.

Economists, professors of anything, engineers, bankers, teachers, company directors and golf course management executives are all of one mind: we must all wear our masks. Astonishingly, and inexplicably, the media is giving yards of print space and many broadcasting hours to these people but denying space or time to experienced, well-qualified doctors who simply want to provide truth, scientific evidence and common sense. The few doctors who toe the 'party line' on the covid-19 hoax are guaranteed huge amounts of publicity.

44.

Will masks become part of the new world religion (widely known to its supporters as Chrislam)?

45.

In a paper published in *MedRxiv.2020* entitled, *Physical interventions to interrupt or reduce the spread of respiratory viruses*, T. Jefferson, M. Jones et al concluded that compared to not wearing a mask there was no reduction of influenza-like illnesses when health care workers or the general population wore masks.
In March 2020, Dr Jenny Harries, Deputy Chief Medical Officer in the UK, warned that it is possible to trap the virus in a mask and start breathing it in. She said that wearing a mask was not a good idea.

46.

A meta-analysis published in May in 2020 by the Centers for Disease Control was entitled, *Non-*

pharmaceutical measures for pandemic influenza in non-healthcare settings – personal protective and environment measures. The authors concluded that the evidence from randomized controlled trials of face masks did not support a substantial effect on the transmission of laboratory-confirmed influenza, either when worn by infected persons or by persons in the general community to reduce their susceptibility.

47.
In May 2016, a meta-analysis written by J. Smith and C. MacDougall and published in the *Canadian Medical Association Journal* concluded that both randomised controlled trials and observational studies of N95 respirators and surgical masks used by health care workers, did not show any benefit against the transmission of acute respiratory infections. The authors also concluded that acute respiratory infection transmission may have occurred via the contamination of provided respiratory protective equipment during storage and through the reuse of masks and respirators during the working day.

48.
In 2019, a scientific paper written by L.Radonovich and M.Simberkoff was published in the *Journal of the American Medical Association*. The paper was entitled, *N95 respirators vs medical masks for preventing influenza among health care personnel: a randomized clinical trial.* The study involved 2,862 volunteers and showed that both surgical masks and N95 respirators

'resulted in no significant difference in the incidence of
laboratory confirmed influenza'.

49.
In 2011, a meta-analysis of 17 separate studies regarding
masks and the effect on the transmission of influenza
found that none of the 17 studies established a
conclusive relationship between mask or respirator use
and protection against influenza infection. The study was
conducted by F. bin-Reza, V. Lopez et al.

50.
It was proved in 1920 that cloth masks fail to impede or
stop flu virus transmissions. It was concluded that the
number of layers of fabric required to prevent pathogen
penetration would require a suffocating number of layers
and could not be used. It was also recognised that there
was a problem of leakage around the edges of cloth
masks.

51.
A paper entitled, *Use of surgical face masks to reduce
the incidence of the common cold among health workers
in Japan: a randomized clinical trial* was published in
the *American Journal of Infection Control* in June 2009.
The authors concluded that face mask use was found not
to be protective against the common cold when
compared to controls who did not wear face masks.

52.

In 2009, investigators studied masks for an article published in the *Journal of Occupational Environmental Hygiene*. The authors concluded that for both N95 masks and surgical masks, expelled particles were deflected around the edges of the masks and that there was measurable penetration of particles through the filter of each mask.

53.

A paper entitled, *Face coverings, aerosol dispersion and mitigation of virus transmission risk*, written by M. Viola, B. Peterson et al, was published in 2005. The authors concluded there have been farther transmissions of virus-laden fluid particles from masked individuals than from unmasked invididuals, by means of leakage jets, including backward and downward jets that may present major hazards. All masks were thought to reduce forward airflow by 90% or more over wearing no mask; however Schlieren imaging showed that surgical masks and cloth masks resulted in a greater upward airflow past the eyebrows than occurred in individuals not wearing masks at all. Backward unfiltered air flow was found to be strong with all the masks tested, compared to individuals not wearing masks. In other words, if a person wearing a mask has an infection then the risk of being infected is high for anyone standing behind the wearer.

54.

A paper by H. Jung and J. Kim, which was entitled, *Comparison of filtration efficiency and pressure drop in anti-yellow sand masks, quarantine masks, medical masks, general masks and handkerchiefs*, was published in *Aerosol Air Qual Res* in June 2013. The paper studied 44 mask brands and found that the average penetration was 35.6%. Even most medical masks had over 20% penetration. Most importantly, the study found that general masks and handkerchiefs had no protective function in terms of aerosol filtration efficiency.

55.

A study published in 2015 in the *British Medical Journal* by C. MacIntyre, H. Seal et al, entitled, *A cluster randomised trial of cloth masks compared with medical masks in healthcare workers* found that penetration of cloth masks by particles was almost 97% while penetration of medical masks was 44%. The authors showed healthcare workers wearing cloth masks had significantly higher rates of influenza-like illness after four weeks of using masks at work – when compared to controls.

56.

It is widely assumed that surgeons and operating theatre staff must wear masks but a paper by N. Mitchell and S. Hunt entitled, *Surgical face masks in modern operating rooms – a costly and unnecessary ritual* which was published in the *Journal of Hospital Infection* in July 1991– found no difference in wound infection rates with and without surgical masks. Other scientific research papers have established similar conclusions. There was, for example, a paper published in 2015 in the *Journal of the Royal Society of Medicine* by C DaZhou, P Sivathondan et al. The paper was entitled, *Unmasking the surgeons: the evidence base behind the use of facemasks in surgery.*

57.

No one should wear a mask while exercising. There have been several reports of masked children dying while exercising. There is evidence showing that mask wearing reduces blood oxygen levels even when the wearer is standing still. Also, individuals who exercise are likely to sweat. Masks then become damp more quickly and the damp promotes the growth of microorganisms.

58.

S. Bae and M. Kim et al published a paper in April 2020 in the journal *Annals Internal Medicine* 2020. The title of their paper was, *Effectiveness of surgical and cotton masks in blocking SARS CoV 2: A controlled comparison in 4 patients* and they concluded that 'neither surgical nor cotton masks effectively filtered SARS-CoV-2 during coughs by infected patients'.

59.

It is not just out of politeness that surgeons and dentists traditionally remove their masks when talking to patients. They do so because they know that patients and relatives find it more reassuring, and more comforting, to

see a whole human face rather than just part of one.
Moreover, it is often exceedingly difficult to understand
what someone is saying when they are wearing a mask.

60.
'The face mask traps warm moisture that is produced
when we exhale,' says dermatologist Dr Maggie Kober.
'For those with acne, this can lead to acne flares. For
many others, this warm, moist environment surrounding
skin creates the perfect condition for naturally occurring
yeast and bacteria to flourish and grow more abundant.
This overgrowth of yeast and bacteria can produce
angular cheilitis, the cracking and sores at the corners of
the mouth.' Face masks can also present a risk of contact
dermatitis and can increase the risk of staph infections.

61.
In June 2020, researchers suggested that the oxygen
reduction and carbon dioxide build up (hypercapnia)
might put a considerable strain on the heart, lungs,
kidneys and immune system. This risk has not been
disproven. The paper was written by B. Chandrasekaran,
S. Fernandes and entitled, *Exercise with facemask: are
we handling a devil's sword – a physiological
hypothesis*.

62.
Research has shown that respirators and masks contained
influenza bugs found on their outer surfaces. The risk
was higher the longer the masks were worn. It has also

been established that bacteria accumulate on masks – and those bacteria can cause lung infections.

63.
Mask wearers are more likely to develop an infection than non-mask wearers. This is most likely to be a result of the wearer breathing in their own heavily contaminated air and, therefore, developing bacterial pneumonia. Infections may also be due to the fact that masks reduce blood oxygen levels and adversely affect natural immunity. It is likely that anyone who wears a face mask for long periods will have a damaged immune system – and be more susceptible to infection. Studies have shown that hypoxia can inhibit immune cells used to fight viral infections. Wearing a mask may make the wearer more likely to develop an infection – and if an infection develops it is likely to be worse. Low oxygen levels reduce T cells and therefore reduce immunity levels.

64.
'Is a mask necessary in the operating theatre?' by N. Orr, published in *Annals Royal College of Surgeons England* in 1981, found no difference in wound infection rates whether or not surgeons wore surgical masks.

65.
Thousands of years ago, it was discovered that forcing people to wear masks covering much of their faces broke their will and made them subservient. The masks depersonalised the wearers and dehumanised them too.

66.

Dr Scott Atlas, White House coronavirus advisor, claimed that face coverings are not effective in stopping the virus's spread. He tweeted, 'Masks work? NO' alongside a link to an article that argued against the success of face coverings. Twitter removed his tweet.

67.

Children are now demanding to be allowed to wear masks (so that they look 'grown up') and some are even fitting masks onto their dolls. Parents do not seem aware that children are especially vulnerable to the brain damage which will inevitably be a result of the hypoxia that is induced by mask wearing.

68.

In some parts of the world (particularly parts of the United States of America) it is compulsory to wear a mask even while exercising. This is particularly dangerous and will lead to a dramatic increase in the number of people dying while exercising.

69.

CIA torture techniques include forcing people to remain isolated (as in lockdowns), to keep their distance from others (social distancing) and to wear masks.

70.

A paper in the journal, *Ophthalmology and Therapy* (published in September 2020), written by Majid Moshirfar, William B. West Jr and Douglas P. Marx

warned of an increase in dry eye symptoms among mask
wearers. Those using masks regularly for extended
periods are more likely to show symptoms. The
condition is caused by exhaled air blowing upwards from
the mask into the eyes. The increased airflow causes
irritation or inflammation. The authors conclude 'this
mask-associated ocular irritation raises concerns about
eye health and increased risk of disease transmission in
prolonged mask users'. Their advice is that lubricant eye
drops should be used and goggles should be worn.
Dry eyes lead to individuals rubbing their eyes which
will lead to an increase in the risk of infection.
Doctors and opticians are also reporting an increase in
the number of patients complaining of persistent
headaches – because of mask wearing.

71.
Those who defend mask wearing claim that the practice
must be safe because surgeons and operating theatre staff
wear masks. But operating theatres are climatically
controlled, masks are replaced every couple of hours,
and those working in an operating theatre do not rush
around doing their shopping. It is important to remember
that surgeons who wear masks (and not all do) work
while standing, rather than walking, and they work in a
controlled, air conditioned environment. They do not
touch their masks and they change them regularly.
Indeed, Physician, Dr J. Meehan MD, who has
performed over 10,000 surgical procedures, has this to
say to those who argue that, 'If masks don't work, then
why do surgeons wear them?'

'Although surgeons do wear masks to prevent their respiratory droplets from contaminating the surgical field and the exposed internal tissues of our surgical patients, that is about as far as the analogy extends…The covid-19 pandemic is about viral transmission. Surgical and cloth masks do nothing to prevent viral transmission. We should all realize by now that face masks have never been shown to prevent or protect against viral transmission. Which is exactly why they have never been recommended for use during the seasonal flu outbreak, epidemics, or previous pandemics. If a surgeon were sick, especially with a viral infection, they would not perform surgery as they know the virus would NOT be stopped by their surgical mask. Another area of "false equivalence" has to do with the environment in which the masks are worn. The environments in which surgeons wear masks minimize the adverse effects surgical masks have on their wearers. Unlike the public wearing masks in the community, surgeons work in sterile surgical suites equipped with heavy duty air exchange systems that maintain positive pressures, exchange and filter the room air at a very high level, and increase the oxygen content of the room air. These conditions limit the negative effects of masks on the surgeon and operating room staff. And yet despite these extreme climate control conditions, clinical studies demonstrate the negative effects (lowering arterial oxygen and carbon dioxide re-breathing) of surgical masks on surgeon physiology and performance. Surgeons and operating room personnel are well trained, experienced, and meticulous about maintaining sterility.

We only wear fresh sterile masks. We don the mask in a sterile fashion. We wear the mask for short periods of time and change it out at the first signs of the excessive moisture build up that we know degrades mask effectiveness and increases their negative effects. Surgeons NEVER re-use surgical masks, nor do we ever wear cloth masks. The public is being told to wear masks for which they have not been trained in the proper techniques. As a result, they are mishandling, frequently touching, and constantly reusing masks in a way that increase contamination and are more likely than not to increase transmission of disease.'

72.
Although the evidence clearly shows that masks do more harm than good, we are told that fines for not wearing masks are going up and the military will be brought in if the police cannot cope.

73.
Mask wearing is making shopping unpleasant, and thereby destroying thousands of small businesses. This is one of the changes in society which will lead to the global reset promoted by the United Nations and its Agenda 21 and the World Economic Forum. The plan is to force us to live in sterile cities and to do all our shopping online.

74.
Mask wearing, social distancing and testing will become a permanent part of our world. The end result will be the

permanent closure of schools – and the moving of education online. Teachers who insist that pupils wear masks and maintain social distancing rules are destroying their own jobs.

75.

A study entitled, *Optical microscopic study of surface morphology and filtering efficiency of face masks* concluded that face masks made of cloth are not very good at filtering out viruses because the pores are much bigger than the particulate matter that needs to be kept out. One study showed that face masks may have pores five thousand times larger than virus particles. This means that the virus will wander through the face mask much like a mouse wandering through Marble Arch.

76.

The World Health Organisation recommends that disposable masks should be discarded after one use. Few people can afford to buy two or more disposable masks for every member of their family, and so masks are frequently worn more than once. This massively increases the risk of a chest infection developing. I predict that in a year or two, there is going to be an epidemic of bacterial pneumonia which is going to be blamed on covid-19 or one of the many mutant strains.

77.

Professor Chris Whitty, the UK's Chief Medical Officer, said in March 2020 that wearing a face mask had almost no effect on reducing the risk of contracting covid-19, and that the Government did not advise healthy individuals to wear masks. Instead, he suggested that people should wash their hands for roughly 20 seconds.

78.
Surgical masks are worn to stop respiratory droplets and human debris from the surgeon or nurse from falling into a wound.

79.
Much of the air we breathe in and out goes around the side of the mask unless it is very tight fitting. Loose fitting masks are therefore entirely useless. Tight fitting masks may provide some filtration protection but the tighter a mask is the greater the risk of serious hypoxia and hypercapnia developing.

80.
It is sometimes said that masks should be worn to protect the elderly, the sick and those with serious health problems. It would make far more sense to suggest to such individuals that they protected themselves from society, if they chose to do so. But they should have the choice. And there is absolutely no reason to force younger, healthy members of society to endure lockdowns (which will clearly kill far more people than covid-19), social distancing (which will create massive psychological problems) or to wear masks (which will do no good but which will cause physical and mental health problems).

81.

A paper published by Boris Borovoy, Collen Huber and Q. Makeeta investigated all types of masks and discovered that 'loose particulate was seen on each type of mask'. They also noted that 'tight and loose fibres were seen on each type of mask' and warned that 'if even a small portion of mask fibres is detachable by inspiratory inflow, or if there is debris in mask manufacture or packaging or handling, then there is the possibility of not only entry of foreign material to the airways but also entry to deep lung tissue, and potential pathological consequences of foreign bodies in the lungs'. The authors draw attention to a correlation between the inhalation of synthetic fibres and various bronchopulmonary diseases such as asthma, alveolitis, chronic bronchitis, bronchiectasis, fibrosis, spontaneous pneumothorax and chronic pneumonia. The authors warn that if widespread masking continues, then the potential for inhaling mask fibres and environmental and biological debris continues on a daily basis for hundreds of millions of people. This should be alarming for physicians and epidemiologists knowledgeable in occupational hazards.' The authors warn that pulmonary fibrosis, a risk of mask wearing, cannot be cured and has a 5 to 20 year survival rate of only 20%.

82.

A mask worn by a child in school was examined in a laboratory. Tests showed 82 bacterial colonies and 4 mould colonies growing on the mask.

83.
'I'm seeing patients that have facial rashes, fungal infections, bacterial infections,' said Dr J. Meehan. 'Reports coming from my colleagues all over the world, are suggesting that the bacterial pneumonias are on the rise. Why might that be? Because untrained members of the public are wearing medical masks, repeatedly in a non-sterile fashion. They're becoming contaminated. They're pulling them off their car seat, off the rear-view mirror, out of their pocket, from their countertop, and they're reapplying a mask that should be worn fresh and sterile every single time.' Dr Meehan also reported an incident where one patient wearing a mask passed out due to low oxygen while at work and fell off a ladder, resulting in serious physical injuries.

84.
If mask wearing were a science, the rules would be constant – but they are not. It is clear, therefore, that there is no science behind mask wearing. Citizens are being forced to wear masks for political reasons.

85.
It is frequently argued that Sweden, which had no lockdown and no mask requirements, has had a very high death rate. If anyone in the media were interested in the facts they would see that the average age of Swedish citizens who died was well over 80, and the great majority of deaths occurred in care homes and nursing homes. The mortality level in Sweden remained below a bad flu season. The Swedish people now seem to have a

high, natural immunity. Fact checkers around the world might like to look at the Imperial College projections, which were alarming, and the actual death rate which was not. Other countries which did not make masks compulsory (such as Japan and some African countries) also had relatively low mortality rates.

86.

A study by M. Walker in 2020 (*MedPage Today* 2020 May 20) found that 624 out of 714 people wearing N95 masks left visible gaps when putting on their masks.

87.

N95 respirators (or masks) are made with a 0.3 micron filter. Their name comes from the fact that 95% of particles having a diameter of 0.3 microns are filtered by the mask. Unfortunately, coronaviruses are approximately 0.125 microns in diameter. Still, these masks will certainly prevent snowballs, flies and other objects getting through.

88.

T. Tunevall wrote a paper called, *Postoperative wound infections and surgical face masks: a controlled study* which was published in the *World Journal Surgery* in 1991. The author reported that the use of masks in surgery was found to slightly increase the incidence of infection over not masking in a study of 3,088 surgeries. The surgeons' masks were found to give no protective effect to the patients.

89.

In the UK, if you don't wear a mask because you have decided you are exempt – and the Government says this is a personal choice – the official advice is that you should not routinely be required to produce any written evidence to justify the fact that you are not wearing a mask. And although I'm no lawyer, I rather doubt that busy bodies, whoever they are, have any right to ask you why you have decided that you are exempt. My website www.vernoncoleman.com includes a link to a section of the Government website which provides an exemption form which can be printed out and attached to a lanyard.

90.

Nine medical authors from Australia and Vietnam studied cloth face masks and concluded that cloth masks should not be recommended for health care workers.

91.

A meta-analysis published in May 2016 concluded that masks did not have any useful effect but that reuse of contaminated masks did transmit infection. Some packs of face masks states that masks do not protect the wearer from the coronavirus.

92.

There is a risk that viruses may accumulate in the fabric of a mask – thereby increasing the amount of the virus being inhaled.

93.

Putting a mask on a baby or an unconscious patient is dangerous. The mask may result in the wearer choking on vomit. In my view, masks on babies could increase the risk of sudden infant death syndrome. No baby should be forced to wear a mask, and yet there are plenty of pictures on the internet showing masks on babies. In some parts of the world, children as young as two are forced to wear masks. Small children are more likely than adults to touch their masks, thereby rendering the masks useless and even more dangerous. Also, small children are more likely to develop a weakened immune system if they wear a mask. Making children wear masks is a form of child abuse.

'It is extremely dangerous to cover a baby's mouth and nose and the design of 'cute' baby face coverings that have been brought to our attention look like they would greatly increase the risk of suffocation. I would strongly advise parents not to use any form of face covering for their baby,' said Dr Rebecca Fletcher, chair of Bury, Rochdale and Oldham Child Death Overview Panel.

94.

Some people claim that face masks give them a sore throat, reports Dr Armando Meza an infectious disease specialist in Texas. 'Humidity will let bacteria continue to grow inside the mask so if you were growing bacteria in that area and you were breathing that inside, you can potentially get an infection, especially strep or any other bacteria that can cause infection.'

95.

In some countries, quite small children are forced to wear masks on transport and even in schools. The evidence supports the view that politicians, teachers and parents who force (or even allow) children to wear masks are guilty of child abuse.

96.

A mask can substantially reduce blood oxygenation – leading to a possible loss of consciousness. At least one road crash has been blamed on a driver wearing a mask. Police reported that the driver of a single car crash in New Jersey, U.S. is believed to have passed out behind the wheel after wearing a mask for too long. Passengers would be wise to avoid travelling in public service vehicles (buses, coaches, etc.) in which the driver is wearing a mask.

97.

Surgeons and nurses are trained never to touch any part of a mask except for the nose bridge and the ear loops. If any part of a mask is touched accidentally then the mask is discarded and replaced.

98.

Over 2,000 Belgian medical professions have urged that covid-19 be prevented by strengthening natural immunity. Their recommendations include specifically to exercise in fresh air without a mask.

99.

A report by Boris Borovoy, Colleen Huber and Maria Crisler reported: 'Masks have been shown through overwhelming clinical evidence to have no effect against transmission of viral pathogens. Penetration of cloth masks by viral particles was almost 97% and of surgical masks was 44%. Even bacteria, approximately ten times the volume of coronaviruses, have been poorly impeded by both cloth masks and disposable surgical masks. After 150 minutes of use, more bacteria were emitted through the disposable mask than from the same subject unmasked. A paper by these authors entitled, *Masks, false safety and real dangers, Part 2: Microbial challenges from masks* is available on the internet and contains a list of 62 scientific journal references showing that masks have no significant preventative impact against any known pathogenic microbes. These authors conclude, 'Specifically, regarding covid-19, we have shown…that mask use is not correlated with lower death rates nor with lower positive PCR tests.' The authors add that, 'Masks have also been demonstrated historically to contribute to increased infections within the respiratory tract' and they conclude that 'the use of face masks will contribute to far more morbidity and mortality than has occurred due to covid-19.'

In their following paper entitled, *Masks false safety and real dangers, Part 3: Hypoxia, hypercapnia and physiological effects* they state: 'In our previous paper in this series, we found a historical correlation with a hypercapnic practice, specifically mask-wearing, and a severe surge of bacterial pneumonia deaths. This time period was mis-named the Spanish Flu, due to a number of reasons, too extensive for this paper. Dr. Anthony Fauci's research team found that every cadaver exhumed form that time in 1918 – 1919 showed the cause of death was bacterial pneumonia, secondary to typical upper respiratory bacteria.' They also go on to say: 'Common and life-threatening diseases of impeded air flow included both obstructive disorders such as asthma, COPD, bronchiectasis and emphysema, as well as restrictive disorders, such as pneumothorax, atelectasis, respiratory distress syndrome and pulmonary fibrosis.'

100.
There is much more evidence supporting the fact that masks should not be worn. Over a dozen scientific papers show clearly that masks are ineffective in preventing the movement of infective organisms and/or reduce oxygen levels, and expose wearers to increased levels of carbon dioxide. Over a dozen studies failed to show that wearing a mask provides protection against infection. In 2011, a meta-analysis of 17 separate studies proved that none of the research showed masks to be useful in preventing influenza infection. The available medical evidence proves overwhelmingly that masks do no good in preventing the spread of infection but do a great deal of harm to those wearing them.

101.
Dr Eric Nepute of St Louis, made a video, which went viral, telling others about what had happened to a four-year-old relative of a patient of his, who nearly died after

developing bacterial pneumonia because of prolonged mask use.

102.

At the University of Witten/Herdecke, Germany, an online registry has been set up where parents, doctors, pedagogues and others can enter their observations. On 20.10.2020, 363 doctors were asked to make entries and to make parents and teachers aware of the registry. By 26.10.2020, the registry had been used by 20,353 people. Parents entered data on a total of 25,930 children. The average wearing time of the mask was 270 minutes per day. Impairments caused by wearing the mask were reported by 68% of the parents. These included irritability (60%), headache (53%), difficulty concentrating (50%), less happiness (49%), reluctance to go to school/kindergarten (44%), malaise (42%), impaired learning (38%) and drowsiness or fatigue (37%).

103.

Kester Disability Rights in the UK helped a disabled woman to win the first face mask discrimination case. The woman was refused access to an unnamed service because she was unable to wear a face mask, and as a result of this egregious discrimination, she was paid £7,000 in compensation. The pay-out was achieved through negotiation as there was no dispute that access had been denied, or that the Claimant had a disability exemption.

104.

In February 21, The North Dakota House of Representatives passed a bill that would prohibit state and local governments, schools and businesses from ordering mask mandates. The bill's sponsor, Rep. Jeff Hoverson who described the rules requiring face masks as 'diabolical silliness' also said, 'The mask is a part of a larger apparatus of a movement of unelected, wealthy bureaucrats, who are robbing our freedoms and perpetuating lies.'

105.

Fifteen million face masks provided to pharmacists in Belgium to be distributed free of charge, caused health chiefs some concern when it was discovered that the face masks might contain nanoparticles of silver and titanium dioxide that when inhaled could lead to pneumonia.

106.

In March 21, a 13-year-old boy was banned from attending classes at the British International School, Stockholm in Danderyd, until he agreed to remove the facemask he was wearing. The public Health Agency of Sweden states, 'Children do not need to wear face masks. It is difficult for children to handle and wear face masks the right way, and children are not the drivers (of infection) in this epidemic and do not spread infection in the same way as adults'.

107.
A recent study in the Journal Cancer Discovery found
that inhalation of harmful microbes can contribute to
advanced stage lung cancer in adults. It is known that
long-term use of face-masks may help breed dangerous
pathogens. Microbiologists agree that frequent mask
wearing creates a perfect, moist environment in which
microbes proliferate before entering the lungs. The
invading microbes travel down the trachea and the
bronchi until they reach the tiny alveoli.
'The lungs were long thought to be sterile, but we now
know that oral commensals – microbes normally found
in the mouth – frequently enter the lungs due to
unconscious aspirations.' – Leopoldo Segal. Study
Author and Director of the Lung Microbiome Program
and Associate Professor of Medicine at New York
University Grossman School of Medicine.
According to the study, after they have invaded the lungs
the microbes cause an inflammatory response in proteins
known as cytokine IL-17.
'Given the known impact of IL-17 and inflammation on
lung cancer. We were interested in determining if the
enrichment of oral commensals in the lungs could drive
an IL-17-type inflammation and influence lung cancer
progression and prognosis,' said Segal.
Whilst analysing lung microbes of 83 untreated adults
with lung cancer, the research team discovered that
colonies of veillonella, prevotella, and streptococcus
bacteria, which may be cultivated through prolonged
mask wearing, are all found in larger quantities in

patients with advanced stage lung cancer than in earlier stages.

The presence of these bacterial cultures is also associated with a lower chance of survival and increased tumour growth regardless of the stage.

108.

Each month, it is estimated that 129 billion face masks and 65 billion gloves are used and disposed of globally. A lot of this waste is ending up in landfills, waterways and oceans, which is having a harmful effect on wildlife - particularly sea life. Non-reusable masks, which are made out of plastics such as polypropylene, take around 450 years to biodegrade, making them just as environmentally unfriendly as plastic carrier bags.

109.

According to the UK Government's website (at the time of writing), the following do not need to wear a face covering:

1) children under the age of 11 (Public Health England does not recommend face coverings for children under the age of 3 for health and safety reasons)

2) people who cannot put on, wear or remove a face covering because of a physical or mental illness or impairment, or disability

3) where putting on, wearing or removing a face covering will cause you severe distress

4) if you are speaking to or providing assistance to someone who relies on lip reading, clear sound or facial expressions to communicate

5) to avoid harm or injury, or the risk of harm or injury, to yourself or others – including if it would negatively impact on your ability to exercise or participate in a strenuous activity
6) police officers and other emergency workers, given that this may interfere with their ability to serve the public.

110.
The UK Government's website has this to say about exemption cards:

If you have an age, health or disability reason for not wearing a face covering:
1) you do not routinely need to show any written evidence of this
2) You do not need to show an exemption card
This means that you do not need to seek advice or request a letter from a medical professional about your reason for not wearing a face covering.
However, some people may feel more comfortable showing something that says they do not have to wear a face covering. This could be in the form of an exemption card, badge or even a home-made sign.
Carrying an exemption card or badge is a person choice and is not required by law.

111.
There is a considerable amount of evidence from around the world to show that politicians who have ordered the public to wear face masks have themselves benefitted

financially. For example, in the UK the National Audit Office found that companies recommended by MPs, peers and ministers' offices were given priority as the Government sought to obtain Personal Protective Equipment.

Conclusion

At no previous time in history have large numbers of people been forced to wear masks. The long-term physical and psychological consequences are unknown though those ordering that masks be worn are no doubt aware of the extraordinary risks and of the way that masks can be used to oppress and subjugate a population. The evidence clearly shows that mask wearing is likely to do no good but a great deal of harm. The big lie, which the WHO, governments everywhere and YouTube want to disseminate, is that wearing masks is essential to control covid-19. But the medical and scientific evidence (banned by YouTube and most mass media) shows that masks have little or no useful effect but can increase the risk of infection and can make breathing difficult. There is little doubt that masks do far more harm than good. Cloth masks are permeable to 97% of viral particles. A study by the University of East Anglia concluded that wearing masks was of no benefit and could increase infection. Experts in respiratory disease and infection protection from the University of Illinois have explained that face masks have no use in everyday life – neither as self-protection nor to protect other people. A study published in the *Annals of Internal Medicine* concluded that neither fabric masks nor surgical masks can prevent the spread of covid-19 by coughing. An article in the *New England Journal of Medicine*, published in May 2020 concluded that masks offer little or no protection and that the call for masks to be compulsory was an irrational fear reflex. A German study showed that masks had no effect on infection rates. Dr Fauci, the American covid-19 supremo, expressed real doubts about masks. On May 28th 2020, he admitted masks are little more than symbolic. Virtue signalling. A meta study on influenza, published in May 2020 by the CDC in America, found that face masks were of no help. The available evidence shows clearly that masks do not work but do have the potential to cause a variety of health problems – including short-term problems such as breathlessness and long-term problems such as brain damage and death. And yet, despite all this, there have been suggestions from various authorities that mask wearing and social distancing will need to be permanent. It has also been suggested that masks should be worn in the home. The sceptical will find it impossible to avoid the conclusion that there is far more to masks (and compulsory mask wearing) than meets the eye.

Afterword

There is absolutely no scientific reason for mask wearing
under any circumstances. The covid-19 hoax is an IQ
test. Anyone who wears a mask after studying the
evidence has clearly failed the test.

Dear Reader

If you found this book useful I would be enormously grateful if you would post a review on social media or your preferred online site. It would help a great deal more than I can tell. And please ask everyone you know to read this book. Thank you

Vernon Coleman

About the Author

Biography and reference articles

Vernon Coleman was educated at Queen Mary's Grammar School in Walsall, Staffs. He then spent a year as a Community Service Volunteer in Liverpool where he was the first of Alec Dickson's 'catalysts'. (Ref 1 below). He studied medicine at Birmingham Medical School and qualified as a doctor in 1970. He has worked both in hospitals and as a GP. He resigned from the health service on a matter of principle. (Ref 2 below). Vernon Coleman has organised many campaigns concerning iatrogenesis, drug addiction and the abuse of animals, and has given evidence to committees at the House of Commons and the House of Lords. For example, he gave evidence to the House of Lords Select Committee on Animals in Scientific Procedures (2001-2) on Tuesday 12.2.02

Dr Coleman's campaigns have often proved successful. For example, after a 15 year campaign (which started in 1973) he eventually persuaded the British Government to introduce stricter controls governing the prescribing of benzodiazepine tranquillisers. ('Dr Vernon Coleman's articles, to which I refer with approval, raised concern about these important matters,' said the Parliamentary Secretary for Health in the House of Commons in 1988.) (Ref 3 below).

Dr Coleman has worked as a columnist for numerous national newspapers including The Sun, The Daily Star, The Sunday Express, Sunday Correspondent and The

People. He once wrote three columns at the same time for national papers (he wrote them under three different names, Dr Duncan Scott in The Sunday People, Dr James in The Sun and Dr Vernon Coleman in the Daily Star). At the same time he was also writing weekly columns for the Evening Times in Glasgow and for the Sunday Scot. His syndicated columns have appeared in over 50 regional newspapers in the United Kingdom and his columns and articles have appeared in newspapers and magazines around the world. Dr Coleman resigned from The People in 2003 when the editor refused to print a column Dr Coleman had written criticising the Government's decision to start the Iraq War. (Ref 6 below)

He has contributed articles and stories to hundreds of other publications including The Sunday Times, Observer, Guardian, Daily Telegraph, Sunday Telegraph, Daily Express, Daily Mail, Mail on Sunday, Daily Mirror, Sunday Mirror, Punch, Woman, Woman's Own, The Lady, Spectator and British Medical Journal. He was the founding editor of the British Clinical Journal. For many years he wrote a monthly newsletter called Dr Vernon Coleman's Health Letter. He has worked with the Open University in the UK and has lectured doctors and nurses on a variety of medical matters.

Vernon Coleman has presented numerous programmes on television and radio and was the original breakfast television doctor on TV AM. He was television's first agony uncle (on BBC1's The Afternoon Show) and presented three TV series based on his bestselling book Bodypower. In the 1980s, he helped write the algorithms for the first computerised health programmes – which sold around the world to those far-sighted individuals who had bought the world's first home computers. (Ref 4 below). His books have been published in the UK by Arrow, Pan, Penguin, Corgi, Mandarin, Star, Piatkus, RKP, Thames and Hudson, Sidgwick and Jackson, Macmillan and many other leading publishing houses and translated into 25 languages. English language versions sell in the USA, Australia, Canada and South Africa as well as the UK. Several of his books have appeared on both the Sunday Times and Bookseller bestseller lists.

Altogether, he has written over 100 books which have, together, sold over two million copies in the UK alone. His self-published novel, Mrs Caldicot's Cabbage War has been turned into an award winning film (starring Pauline Collins, John Alderton and Peter Capaldi) and the book is, like many of his other novels, available in an audio version.

Vernon Coleman has co-written five books with his wife, Donna Antoinette Coleman, and has, in addition, written numerous articles (and books) under a vast variety of pennames (many of which he has now forgotten). Donna Antoinette Coleman is a talented oil painter who specialises in landscapes. Her books include, My Quirky Cotswold Garden. She is a Fellow of the Royal Society of Arts. Vernon and Antoinette Coleman have been married for more than 20 years.

Vernon Coleman has received numerous awards and was for some time a Professor of Holistic Medical Sciences at the Open International University based in Sri Lanka.

Reference Articles referring to Vernon Coleman

Ref 1

'Volunteer for Kirkby' – The Guardian, 14.5.1965
(Article re VC's work in Kirkby, Liverpool as a
Community Service Volunteer in 1964-5)

Ref 2

'Bumbledom forced me to leave the NHS' – Pulse,
28.11.1981
(Vernon Coleman resigns as a GP after refusing to
disclose confidential information on sick note forms)

Ref 3

'I'm Addicted To The Star' – The Star, 10.3.1988

Ref 4

'Medicine Becomes Computerised: Plug In Your
Doctor.' – The Times, 29.3.1983

Ref 5

'Computer aided decision making in medicine' – British
Medical Journal, 8.9.1984 and 27.10.1984

Ref 6

'Conscientious Objectors' – Financial Times magazine,
9.8.2003

Major interviews with Vernon Coleman include

'Doctor with the Common Touch.' – Birmingham Post,
9.10.1984

'Sacred Cows Beware: Vernon Coleman publishing
again.' – The Scotsman, 6.12.1984

'Our Doctor Coleman Is Mustard' – The Sun, 29.6.1988

'Reading the mind between the lines.' – BMA News
Review, November 1991

'Doctors' Firsts' – BMA News Review, 21.2.1996
'The big league of self publishing.' – Daily Telegraph, 17.8.1996
'Doctoring the books' – Independent, 16.3.1999
'Sick Practices' – Ode Magazine, July/August 2003
'You have been warned, Mr Blair.' – Spectator, 6.3.2004 and 20.3.2004
'Food for thought with a real live Maverick.' – Western Daily Press, 5.9.2006
'The doctor will see you now' – Independent, 14.5.2008

There is a more comprehensive list of reference articles on www.vernoncoleman.com

The Author

Dr Vernon Coleman MB ChB DSc was the first qualified medical practitioner in the UK to question the significance of the 'crisis' now described as covid-19, telling readers of his website www.vernoncoleman.com at the end of February 2020 that he felt that the team advising the Government had been unduly pessimistic and had exaggerated the danger of the virus. At the beginning of March, he explained how and why the mortality figures had been distorted. And on March 14th, he warned that the Government's policies would result in far more deaths than the disease itself. In a YouTube video recorded on 18th March, he explained his fear that the Government would use the 'crisis' to oppress the elderly and to introduce compulsory vaccination. And he revealed on his website and in subsequent videos that the infection had been downgraded on March 19th 2020 when the public health bodies in the UK and the Advisory Committee on Dangerous Pathogens decided that the 'crisis' infection should no longer be classified as a 'high consequence infectious disease'. Just days after the significance of the infection had been officially downgraded, the Government published an Emergency Bill which gave the police extraordinary new powers and put millions of people under house arrest. Dr Coleman, a former GP principal, is a *Sunday Times* bestselling author. His books have sold over two million copies in the UK, been translated into 25 languages and sold all around the world. He has given evidence to the House of Commons and the House of Lords, and his campaigning has changed Government policy. There is a short biography at the back of this book. Some references have been given in this book in view of the misleading information widely available online as part of the demonization process now being used to attack those questioning the 'official' line. Vernon Coleman's first book about the coronavirus, *Coming Apocalypse*, was only accepted for publication after all specific references to coronavirus and covid-19 were removed. (Careful editing worked in alternative words and phrases.) Vernon Coleman's second book about the coronavirus hoax (a collection of the transcripts of the videos broadcast between April and September) was titled, *Covid-19: The Greatest Hoax in History*. The book was banned within days of publication. A second version of the same book titled, *Old Man in a Chair* was banned within hours of publication. Vernon Coleman then published an eBook version of *Old Man in a Chair* on Smashwords, unfortunately, this too was banned.

'Vernon Coleman writes brilliant books.' – The Good Book Guide

'No thinking person can ignore him.' – The Ecologist

'The calmest voice of reason.' – The Observer

'A godsend.' – Daily Telegraph

'Superstar.' – Independent on Sunday

'Brilliant!' – The People

'Compulsive reading.' – The Guardian

'His message is important.' – The Economist

'He's the Lone Ranger, Robin Hood and the Equalizer rolled into one.' – Glasgow Evening Times

'The man is a national treasure.' – What Doctors Don't Tell You

'His advice is optimistic and enthusiastic.' – British Medical Journal

'Revered guru of medicine.' – Nursing Times

'Gentle, kind and caring' – Western Daily Press

'His trademark is that he doesn't mince words. Far funnier than the usual tone of soupy piety you get from his colleagues.' – The Guardian

'Dr Coleman is one of our most enlightened, trenchant and sensitive dispensers of medical advice.' – The Observer

'I would much rather spend an evening in his company than be trapped for five minutes in a radio commentary box with Mr Geoffrey Boycott.' – Peter Tinniswood, Punch

'Hard hitting...inimitably forthright.' – Hull Daily Mail

'Refreshingly forthright.' – Liverpool Daily Post

'Outspoken and alert.' – Sunday Express

'Dr Coleman made me think again.' – BBC World Service

'Marvellously succinct, refreshingly sensible.' – The Spectator

'Probably one of the most brilliant men alive today.' – Irish Times

'King of the media docs.' – The Independent

'Britain's leading medical author.' – The Star

'Britain's leading health care campaigner.' – The Sun

'Perhaps the best known health writer for the general public in the world today.' – The Therapist

'The patient's champion.' – Birmingham Post

'A persuasive writer whose arguments, based on research and experience, are sound.' – Nursing Standard

'The doctor who dares to speak his mind.' – Oxford Mail

'He writes lucidly and wittily.' – Good Housekeeping

Books by Vernon Coleman include:

Medical
The Medicine Men
Paper Doctors
Everything You Want To Know About Ageing
The Home Pharmacy
Aspirin or Ambulance
Face Values
Stress and Your Stomach
A Guide to Child Health
Guilt
The Good Medicine Guide
An A to Z of Women's Problems
Bodypower
Bodysense
Taking Care of Your Skin
Life without Tranquillisers
High Blood Pressure
Diabetes
Arthritis
Eczema and Dermatitis
The Story of Medicine
Natural Pain Control
Mindpower
Addicts and Addictions
Dr Vernon Coleman's Guide to Alternative Medicine
Stress Management Techniques
Overcoming Stress
The Health Scandal
The 20 Minute Health Check

Sex for Everyone
Mind over Body
Eat Green Lose Weight
Why Doctors Do More Harm Than Good
The Drugs Myth
Complete Guide to Sex
How to Conquer Backache
How to Conquer Pain
Betrayal of Trust
Know Your Drugs
Food for Thought
The Traditional Home Doctor
Relief from IBS
The Parent's Handbook
Men in Bras, Panties and Dresses
Power over Cancer
How to Conquer Arthritis
How to Stop Your Doctor Killing You
Superbody
Stomach Problems – Relief at Last
How to Overcome Guilt
How to Live Longer
Coleman's Laws
Millions of Alzheimer Patients Have Been Misdiagnosed
Climbing Trees at 112
Is Your Health Written in the Stars?
The Kick-Ass A–Z for over 60s
Briefs Encounter
The Benzos Story
Dementia Myth

Psychology/Sociology
Stress Control
How to Overcome Toxic Stress
Know Yourself (1988)
Stress and Relaxation
People Watching
Spiritpower
Toxic Stress
I Hope Your Penis Shrivels Up
Oral Sex: Bad Taste and Hard To Swallow
Other People's Problems
The 100 Sexiest, Craziest, Most Outrageous Agony
Column Questions (and Answers) Of All Time
How to Relax and Overcome Stress
Too Sexy To Print
Psychiatry
Are You Living With a Psychopath?

Politics and General
England Our England
Rogue Nation
Confronting the Global Bully
Saving England
Why Everything Is Going To Get Worse Before It Gets
Better
The Truth They Won't Tell You...About The EU
Living In a Fascist Country
How to Protect & Preserve Your Freedom, Identity &
Privacy
Oil Apocalypse
Gordon is a Moron

Why Is Public Hair Curly
People Push Bottles Up Peaceniks
Secrets of Paris
Moneypower
101 Things I Have Learned
100 Greatest Englishmen and Englishwomen
Cheese Rolling, Shin Kicking and Ugly Tattoos
One Thing after Another

Novels (General)
Mrs Caldicot's Cabbage War
Mrs Caldicot's Knickerbocker Glory
Mrs Caldicot's Oyster Parade
Mrs Caldicot's Turkish Delight
Deadline
Second Chance
Tunnel
Mr Henry Mulligan
The Truth Kills
Revolt
My Secret Years with Elvis
Balancing the Books
Doctor in Paris
Stories with a Twist in the Tale (short stories)
Dr Bullock's Annals

The Young Country Doctor Series
Bilbury Chronicles
Bilbury Grange
Bilbury Revels
Bilbury Country

Bilbury Village
Bilbury Pie (short stories)
Bilbury Pudding (short stories)
Bilbury Tonic
Bilbury Relish
Bilbury Mixture
Bilbury Delights
Bilbury Joys
Bilbury Tales
Bilbury Days
Bilbury Memories

Novels (Sport)
Thomas Winsden's Cricketing Almanack
Diary of a Cricket Lover
The Village Cricket Tour
The Man Who Inherited a Golf Course
Around the Wicket
Too Many Clubs and Not Enough Balls

Cat books
Alice's Diary
Alice's Adventures
We Love Cats
Cats Own Annual
The Secret Lives of Cats
Cat Basket
The Cataholics' Handbook
Cat Fables
Cat Tales
Catoons from Catland

As Edward Vernon
Practice Makes Perfect
Practise What You Preach
Getting Into Practice
Aphrodisiacs – An Owner's Manual
The Complete Guide to Life

Written with Donna Antoinette Coleman
How to Conquer Health Problems between Ages 50 & 120
Health Secrets Doctors Share With Their Families
Animal Miscellany
England's Glory
Wisdom of Animals